Build

Immune Resilience

A Scientific and Actionable Approach to Upgrade Your Body's Core Defense System

immuneresilience.com

Amit Sood, MD MSc FACP

Happier Stronger Kinder

ISBN 13: 978-1-7347377-0-7
Imprint Name: Global Center for Resiliency and Wellbeing,
Rochester, MN

Disclaimer

The information in this book is not intended to substitute a health care provider's advice or medical care. Please consult your physician or other health care provider if you are experiencing any symptoms or have questions pertaining to the information contained in this book.

Faced with a threat or uncertainty, you have two options:

#1. It is what it is. I can't do much about it; I will wait and see what happens. Or worse, I will let my fear paralyze me.

#2. I don't accept inaction. I can do a lot. I won't let fear grip me, will take charge, and maximize my chances of defeating this threat.

I like the second option much better.

I believe one of the most important things you and I can do to face our current challenge is to bolster our resilience, particularly immune resilience.

A strong and intelligent immune system will not only help you better face today's challenge, but it will make you stronger for any future such threats that might knock at your door.

Dear friends,

Adversities can put our brain in a "worry mode" or a "think and act mode." Like you, I am concerned about the ongoing epidemic. But I realize that my "worry mode" won't help. I want to think and act.

With effective vaccines and antivirals not presently available, many are asking, *"Beyond hand hygiene, social distancing, disinfecting the surfaces, and following the news, what else can I do to take care of myself?"* Here are some of my thoughts. Most are based on peer-reviewed research, that although not always conclusive, is compelling enough to implement a few self-care strategies.

****

Every infection is a battle between the pathogen and the host's immune system. Quite simply, the outcome of infection can be:

A. Complete recovery
B. Overwhelming infection
C. Overwhelming inflammation

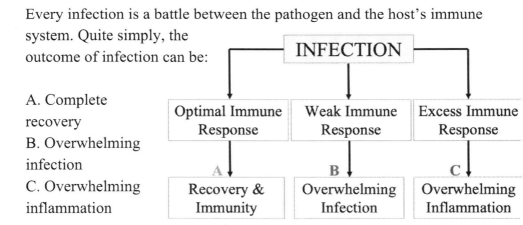

A is your most likely outcome, which is a comforting thought. Nevertheless, for some, B happens, often when they have a weak immune system (from chronic illness, extremes of age, etc.).

A few might experience C because of an overly vigorous immune response. Occasionally, you can have a weak immune system that also produces overwhelming inflammation—a combination of B and C.

How do you increase the chances of experiencing A? Allow me to introduce to you the concept of **immune resilience**. **A resilient immune system mounts an optimal innate and adaptive response, without causing excessive inflammation**.

Literature, that in many instances is provocative but not conclusive, supports the following 15 ideas to strengthen your immune response while limiting inflammation. They are:

1. Correct micronutrient deficiency
2. Get adequate sleep
3. Do moderate physical activity
4. Manage my stress better
5. Build emotional resilience
6. Practice meditation or another mind-body practice
7. Feel socially connected / Improve relationships
8. Invest time in a personally meaningful spiritual practice
9. Nurture hope
10. Laugh more
11. Get a massage
12. Add music to my life
13. Stop smoking
14. Decrease alcohol intake
15. Consider taking a supplement

Correct micronutrient deficiency – Micronutrients include vitamins A, B2, B6, B12, folic acid, C, D, and E, iron, selenium, copper, and zinc. While the best source of micronutrients is a healthy diet, if you are a vegan, have dietary restrictions or malabsorption, or otherwise limited in your food intake, taking a supplement might help. If you think you don't lack in one or more of the micronutrients, remember that per CDC, globally, almost two billion people are micronutrient deficient.

Get adequate sleep – About 50 percent of us aren't getting adequate sleep. Fairly conclusive research supports the immune-suppressive and inflammatory effect of sleep deficit. Prioritize getting good seven hours, particularly during times when you need a resilient immune system to protect you. Commit to a discipline, and if your sleep isn't restorative, consider seeing a specialist.

Do moderate physical activity – For your immunity, physical activity in moderation is better than a sedentary lifestyle or (perhaps) very vigorous exercise. Do something, however little, and remain agile during the day. Consider Yoga and Tai Chi, that have independently shown anti-inflammatory and immune-enhancing effects.

Manage your stress better – Excessive stress is a pro-inflammatory state and weakens your immune system. Consider creating a "Not-to-do list" to give a haircut to your cognitive and emotional load. Cultivate self-compassion by letting go of perfectionism and believing in those who believe in you.

Build resilience – Resilience is the core strength you use to lift the load of life. Cultivate a stronger attention and build a resilient mindset using the five principles of gratitude, compassion, acceptance, meaning, and forgiveness.

Practice meditation or another mind-body practice – Several studies have demonstrated that practicing meditation lowers inflammatory molecules and enhances your NK cell activity that help with the anti-viral response. Further, meditation may also help with the antibody response to vaccination. Invest at least 10 minutes a day practicing deep breathing or another form of meditation.

Feel socially connected – Perceived loneliness hurts our immune system. The less lonely and more connected you feel, the better your immunity and less your propensity to inflammation. Minimize adversarial connections by cultivating kindness. Think of someone you may have been wanting to forgive for a long time. Now is the time to make it real.

Practice a personally meaningful spiritual activity – Practicing spirituality (faith-based or secular) correlates with lower levels of inflammatory markers, in both observational and prospective studies. This is a great time to think about what matters most to you and engage with it.

Nurture hope – Hope has a broad effect on your wellbeing, including on your immune system. The more you feel connected to others, think about the beautiful past, focus on your life's purpose, and invest in self-care, the more hopeful you will feel.

Laugh more – Laughter is a great mini workout for your body, improving your immunity and decreasing your inflammatory response. Spend time with people who make you laugh, watch funny videos, read books that make you giggle, and create your personal humor. Remember to laugh with and not laugh at.

Get a massage – You will be surprised how many studies have looked at the health (and immune) benefits of massage. Take time to pamper yourself with a professional or do self-massage.

Add music to your life – Music can reverse the harmful effects of stress on your immune system. Music that adds social connection, such as choir, drumming, and others, can be especially beneficial. Add music to your day as a background, and if you have the time, spend some committed moments savoring your favorite music.

Stop smoking – This is a no brainer, and I won't belabor it here except for saying that smoking wreaks havoc on your immune system, predisposing you to pneumonia and other infections.[1]

Avoid excessive alcohol – If you binge five times a month, it's time to scale that down. While mild to moderate alcohol intake may not hurt your immune system, heavy alcohol intake is definitely harmful.

Consider select supplements – I have mixed feelings about this topic. While I am intrigued by the idea of bovine colostrum and echinacea, the data isn't conclusive to support their intake. Consider adding a few ingredients such as blueberries, grapes, broccoli, garlic, ginger, probiotics, and turmeric to your diet, and correcting any micronutrient deficiency.

****

No doubt, the most essential part of protecting yourself is appropriate preventive actions, particularly hand hygiene. Be uptodate on your immunizations also. The following two links provide comprehensive and up to date information about the preventive approaches:
https://www.cdc.gov/coronavirus/2019-ncov/index.html
https://www.who.int/emergencies/diseases/novel-coronavirus-2019

But with effective vaccines and antivirals about a year away, is there something else you and I can do to help ourselves? I believe the answer is a definite yes. Instead of letting your brain stew in the worry mode, this is a good time to enhance your emotional and physical resilience, particularly immune resilience.

I hope and pray that the current epidemic doesn't reach your backyard, but if it does, I pray you and your loved ones experience it as an ordinary cold and nothing more.

Take care.

Amit
March 2nd, 2020

Immunity Matters

It's 1901. The commonest causes of mortality are pneumonia, influenza, tuberculosis, and gastro-intestinal infections.[2] Diphtheria, typhoid, and smallpox are dreaded names. Alexander Fleming is only 20 years old and a private in the London Scottish Regiment of the Volunteer Force. The first antibiotic is almost three decades away. Cancer is an inconsequential, almost unheard-of name.

Fast forward now to 2020. So much has changed. We have eliminated smallpox, and markedly controlled measles, diphtheria, tetanus, polio, and more. Chronic illnesses have taken the forefront with 70 percent of us having one or another chronic illness. But, partly because of our mistakes, we are facing newer infections for which we have little natural defense and limited to no drug treatments. Some of these infections spread fast and have the potential to invade deeper in the body, particularly in the elderly and the frail.

The present epidemic has created an international crisis with considerable concern that this could become a once in a century pandemic.[3] Our natural response to the barrage of negative headline news is fear. But fear is precisely what you don't need in these times. Let me tell you why.

Tuberculosis mortality was very high in the Western Europe in the 1800. But then it started declining steeply so that by 1950 mortality from TB was about 95 percent lower. **All of this drop in mortality happened before the first medication to treat TB (Streptomycin) was introduced.** In other words—TB mortality came down not because of

> The greatest drop in mortality from tuberculosis happened before the discovery of antibiotics.

an effective medicine, but because of something else. That something else was hygiene and nutrition.[4] Let's see how it played out.

The fight with the bacteria and viruses has two sides to the equation—the virulence of the pathogen (bacteria, viruses, fungi, etc.) and the immunity of the host. **The virulence of the pathogen may not be in your control, but you have tremendous influence on your immunity. Immunity matters.**

The same flu virus can be an annoying few days of fever or take you to the ICU, or worse. In almost every study, an age above 65 is a predictor of an adverse outcome, as are chronic illnesses such as heart, kidney, liver or lung disease, cancer, and diabetes. Interestingly, high level of stress is also a predictor of an adverse outcome.[5] **Each of these predictors operate through one mechanism—weakening your immune system.**

> The same flu can be an annoying few days of fever or a life-threatening infection. A lot depends on your immune response.

Unlike the pre-antibiotic pre-vaccine era, we now depend a lot on immunization and antibiotics to fight the pathogens. Both of these are extremely helpful, but not of much value for many viruses and bacteria against which we have no vaccines or antibiotics.

Because of this overreliance, we haven't prioritized building a resilient immune system, one that strongly responds to the invading agents, yet at the same time doesn't produce unnecessary inflammation. That's precisely what we need today.

Further, as I will soon share in the research studies cited, **we have hurt our immune system with many of the modern lifestyle choices we have made.**

The current epidemic is a rude awakening. We definitely need to build a robust healthcare system and international collaboration to prevent, detect, and better handle such epidemics.[3] Simultaneously, each of us must develop a resilient body and a resilient immune system that give a tough fight to invading pathogens.

Presently, we all will be helped by a two-pronged approach:
1. **Implement rational preventive approaches (as outlined by the CDC and other agencies).**
2. **Build a resilient immune system.**

In this book I share the science and art of developing a resilient immune system.

Note: Please read this book concurrent with the writings, videos and other content on the website *immuneresilience.com*.

Contents

1. What is Immune Resilience?

The word immune means protection. In the context of your immune system, it confers protection from infections. Although the immune system helps you in many different ways including protection from cancer, healing wounds, and more, in this book our focus is on the immune system's role in fighting and preventing infections.

The challenge

Every life form invests significant resources protecting itself from other life forms. For the threats from large predators, our muscles, the nervous system, the cardiovascular system, and the endocrine system coordinate to fight the predator or run away. But how do you handle a threat that presents itself as a sore throat caused by billions of nanometer size particles? That threat has to be handled at the microscopic level with nanometer sized bullets. That's the job of our immune system.

Here are the four-pronged challenge our immune system faces:
- **Attack the pathogens**
- **Not attack the friendly bacteria (such as the colonic microbiome)**
- **Minimize damage to our own body**
- **Deal with constantly changing threat**

A resilient immune system attacks and eliminates the actual threat, without hurting its own body or the friendly bacteria, inflicts only the

> A resilient immune system is not only strong, it is specific, controlled, and adaptive.

necessary amount of damage, and adapts to the everchanging threats. In other words, it is **potent, specific, controlled, and adaptive**. Let's look at each one of these attributes.

1. Potent

Imagine walking in the dark of the night in the woods not knowing from where a predator can lunge. You will do two things: Be preemptively agile wearing a protective gear and act decisively to neutralize the threat if it materializes. Since you don't know what kind of threat might come from where, your pre-emptive agility is nonspecific and always active, while your actions to neutralize the materialized threat are specific and situational. The immune system operates the same way in two highly integrated compartments—the innate system and the adaptive system.

The innate system. Your innate immune system responds to a broad set of threats. Intact skin and mucosa, the mucus layer, moving cilia, molecules in the mucus (complement proteins, defensins, cytokines, chemokines, enzymes, and others)—they are all the first line of defense. They prevent the entry of the pathogen past your body's gates.

If the pathogen sneaks its way in, it meets an army of cells—neutrophils, mast cells, basophils, eosinophils, monocytes, dendritic cells, macrophages, natural killer (NK) cells. They recognize molecular patterns in the pathogen, poke holes and shoot toxic enzymes and chemicals to inflict direct damage. A number of chemicals—antibodies, complement, interferon, interleukins, and more support this process. While the system has redundancies, each arm of the system has its own niche. Deficits in NK cell activity causes unique infections (particularly the viral infections e.g. herpes virus), while complement deficit causes pneumonias and abscesses.

> For many novel threats, the innate immune system is your first line of defense.

The moment your innate system perceives a threat, it effects the release of chemicals to increase blood flow and produce inflammation. Further, this system alerts the second response—the adaptive system.

The adaptive system
While the innate system is broad and nonspecific, the adaptive system is focused and specific. It needs considerable resources and so it is launched only once your body has recognized the threat and it is deemed serious. That makes it slow.

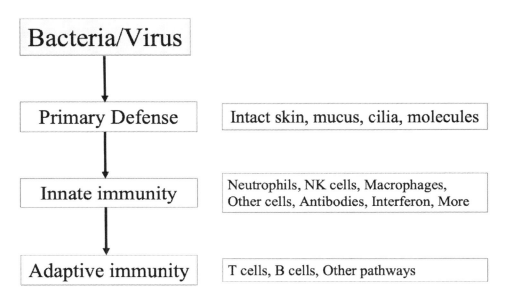

The adaptive system is made of a specific type of cells called the lymphocytes. The lymphocytes are of two types—the B cells and the T cells. Each of these cells have receptors on their surface to recognize different types of microbes. Once a cell in the innate system (such as the macrophage), presents the information to the lymphocytes that have receptors that match with the protein on the cell (the antigen), the lymphocytes are activated. They multiply and disperse, inform other parts of the immune system, and unleash injury to the pathogen.

Each type of cells has a unique function. B cells make antibodies and present information to the T cells. Antibodies coat the microbe, stopping it in its tracks, mark the microbe to be killed by other cells, and activate other pathways such as the complement. Different types of T cells help the B cells with antibody production (CD4 cells) and directly kill the microbe (CD8 cells). They also attract

> The adaptive immune system is specific, focused, and strong, but is often slow.

the innate cells (neutrophils and macrophages) and regulate the intensity of the immune response.

The above description is by no means comprehensive, but I hope gives you an idea about its complexity and richness.

2. Specific

No army wishes to kill its own soldiers in friendly fire. The same applies to the immune system. Our immune system has enough chemicals to kill and digest our body in a very short time. But that doesn't happen because we have elaborate ways to parse self from not self.

The key step here is recognizing the protein signature. Danger and pathogens have specific molecular patterns (called the danger or pathogen associated molecular patterns—DAMP or PAMP). Once the innate immune response recognizes this pattern, it directs its soldiers to eliminate the source of these patterns. The normal body cells do not have this protein signature and thus remain safe.

In the adaptive immunity, cells that produce antibodies with poor affinity to the antigen are destroyed. This ensures that the antibodies are target specific. Even in early processing, only the cells that are likely to recognize the self from non self enter the circulation.

3. Controlled

You may have heard of the term, surgical strike. In this instance a coordinated military attack neutralizes a legitimate target with minimal damage to surrounding structures. One version of this is precision bombing. While, we wish to live in a world with no strike and no bombing, surgical strike and precision bombing are perhaps better than a full-scale war and carpet bombing.

Your immune system has multiple checks and balances to make sure it inflicts only the damage necessary to neutralize the threat. It constantly destroys its own cells that don't seem well trained (i.e. not locked on the right antigen). It also has cells committed to unleash a negative feedback loop that slow the assault.

4. Adaptive

Most body organs do the same job every single day. But not the immune system. **Our immune system faces novel threats on most days.** One day it might be fighting a virus, another day healing a scar, and a third day killing a rogue cancer cell. Never a dull moment for the immune system, given that millions of potential threats work against us, several unknown and continuously evolving. Most bacteria and viruses are much nimbler replicating several times faster than our body cells. The immune system thus has to work like a startup company, even though it is a large, complex, and a very old conglomerate.

> Your immune system keeps you safe from novel threats every single day.

An interesting mechanism by which your immune system accomplishes flexibility is by creating millions of different receptor types through a process called genetic recombination. Through a random process, our system constantly generates novel receptors, in the hope that if we face a new threat, we will have at least a few cells that can start the process of neutralization. Our system is thus constantly on the move, playing catch up with the pathogens that themselves are on the move.

In most situations for people born with good health, this system with its attributes of potency, specificity, control, and adaptiveness, keeps you safe and healthy. But not infrequently, the system crumbles, particularly if we do little to keep it strong, or worse, lead a life that hurts our immune resilience. That's where we are going next, after touching upon one more aspect of the immune system—it's phenomenal memory.

Phenomenal memory

Your immune system is easy to take an offence and doesn't forget its insults. And that's a good thing.

Once the adaptive arm of your immune system activates, it keeps that experience in its memory. This is in the form of cells that are committed to respond to a specific protein signature (memory cells). The body also manufactures antibodies that circulate in your blood and lymph and are secreted in the mucosa.

Vaccination relies on this principle. By giving you a subdued form of the pathogen or a protein that elicits the immune response, your health care providers hope to confer you the protection without causing the illness. This process educates and prepares the immune system.

****

Here is the bottom line: We are born with an immune system that is strong, careful, flexible, and intelligent. It defends us every single day from countless threats. It is ready and armed to protect us. But here is the question I ask: **Won't it be right for us to play our part in keeping our immune system resilient?**

> Your immune system is your invisible tool that is ever ready to fight on your side.

Unfortunately, we may be wanting a bit in that effort. Let me spend a few moments introducing you to some of our habits that hurt our immune system. We will then move to the central theme of our discussion—ways to develop immune resilience.

2. Why We Lose Immune Resilience?

Vultures dine on carcass that may have been rotting for days. Dogs take refreshing gulps out of the toilet bowl, bears love to ravage the garbage cans, alligators swim in marshy waters. Yet, they all do okay. This is because they all have uniquely resilient immune systems adapted to their lifestyle. For example, vultures have very strong acid in their stomach that can digest ingested bone.

Our immune system is also inherently strong. That's how we have survived the plague and flu pandemics of the past. But of late, our lifestyle is slowly hurting our immune resilience. An immune system that loses its potency, specificity, control, and adaptive nature predisposes its host to uncontrolled infections, auto-immune conditions, and inflammation. Here is a list of some of our lifestyle choices that can hurt our immune system:

> Many of our lifestyle choices are weakening our immune system. But we can reverse this by making better choices.

- Micronutrient deficiency
- Sleep deficiency or non-restorative sleep
- Excessive caloric intake
- Sedentary lifestyle
- Psychological stress
- Perceived loneliness
- Cigarette smoking
- Excessive alcohol intake
- Addiction to drugs

All of the above predispose to chronic illness, which may indeed be a product of unhealthy immune system.

In general, when you tell your immune system I am planning on staying on this planet for a long time, your immune system obliges by planning to keep you safe and not inflamed. **If, however, you show apathy toward your wellbeing, your immune system also becomes apathetic.**

The next six chapters are devoted to a systematic approach to build immune resilience.

3. Correct Two Deficits

The modern lifestyle produces two important deficits—that of micronutrients and sleep.

Micronutrient deficit

Two important questions

What are micronutrients?
Am I getting enough micronutrients?

The science:

Micronutrients are dietary components that are essential for development, disease prevention, and wellbeing, even though we need them in small amounts. They include the vitamins and minerals (vitamins A, B2, B6, and B12, folic acid, C, D, E, iron, selenium, copper, and zinc). **We need to take them from outside sources since our body cannot produce any of the micronutrients.** Unfortunately, we often lack these essential chemicals. Globally, per the CDC, almost

> Almost a third of the world's population suffers from micronutrient deficiency.

two billion people have micronutrient deficiency.

Micronutrient deficiency weakens the immune system and predisposes to inflammation.[6] The deficiencies affect both the skin and mucosal barriers, innate immunity, and the adaptive response (T cell and B cell responses).[7] For example, vitamins A, C, E and zinc help keep your skin intact and healthy, while vitamins A, B6, B12, C, D, E, and folic acid help the maturation of the immune cells. Vitamins C, E, selenium, copper, and zinc neutralize the damage by reactive oxygen species to the immune cells.[8] Almost all of the micronutrients are essential for antibody production. The deficiencies thus result in recurrent and chronic infections.[9]

The infections by themselves predispose to micronutrient deficiencies by decreasing intake, increasing losses, and impairing micronutrient utilization.[7] This can set up a harmful feedback loop.

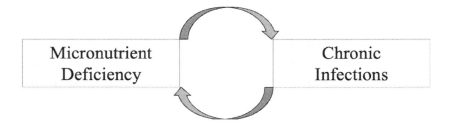

Micronutrient Deficiency — Chronic Infections

Given that these deficiencies are more common in people with chronic illness, alcohol abuse, and weakened immune system, it's obvious that micronutrient deficiency affects and hurts the most vulnerable. Micronutrient deficiency may be one reason people with chronic illnesses experience worse outcomes from infections.

Even marginal micronutrient deficiency can impair the immune system.[10] Further, micronutrient supplementation has been shown to improve the immune system and decrease the risk of infections.[11] Supplementation also decreases the inflammatory immune response. [8,12]

> Micronutrient supplementation can decrease the risk of infections and contain inflammation by improving the immune system.

At the other extreme of micronutrient deficiency is macronutrient excess, particularly of refined sugars and low-quality fat.

Excessive caloric intake and the associated weight gain predisposes to inflammation,[13] poor coordination between the innate and adaptive immune responses, and disruption of the lymphoid tissue, predisposing you to infections.[14] Excessive weight gain increases your risk of worse outcomes from influenza.[15]

Further, **the immune changes also hamper your response to vaccination**. You want to give your immune system the best chance to respond to the vaccines given to you. Otherwise you have invited the side effects, without the benefit.[14]

Suggested actions:

Here are three suggested actions to correct your micronutrient deficiency and macronutrient excess:

- **Eat smart**
- **Eat fewer calories**
- **Consider taking a supplement**

Eat smart: Since micronutrients are present in a variety of food items, eat different types of food. Whenever possible eat fresh. Emphasize fresh fruits, vegetables, nuts, legumes, eggs, fish, and other healthy foods.

Several studies have shown that **higher intake of fruits and vegetables improves immunity, and lowers inflammation and oxidative stress**.[16,17] Interestingly, positive effects are seen not only with whole fruits, but also with juice concentrates and powders.[18,19]

Also, consider adding spices to your food. Spices like turmeric, coriander, ginger, cinnamon, cayenne, and black pepper provide excellent antioxidant effect which may curb inflammation.[20,21]

Eat fewer calories: Perhaps you have been wanting to tame your caloric intake for some time. If that's the case, now is the right time—in the interest of your immune system. **You may not have to decrease the total amount of food you eat; just enhance its quality. Prioritize low calorie dense options.** You can also consider intermittent fasting, that is showing interesting beneficial effects on the immune system in some of the early studies.[22,23]

Consider taking a supplement: If you have known deficiency, a chronic condition that can be worsened by a deficiency or are limited in the variety of foods you can eat, then consider taking a micronutrient supplement. If you choose to take a supplement, avoid the ones that provide excessive amounts of vitamins and minerals. Instead, choose the ones that provide close to a 100

> Avoid taking supplements that provide excessive dose of particular micronutrients.

percent of recommended daily intake. I generally suggest taking these supplements two to three times a week. Check with your physician if this is OK for you, particularly to make sure that the supplements you take doesn't interact with any of your other medications or medical condition.

Sleep deficit

Two important questions

Am I getting sufficient sleep?
Is my sleep of good quality?

The Science:

Between 30 to 40 percent of us do not get sufficient sleep (7 or more hours in the night), and between 10 to 20 percent experience non-restorative sleep.[24] **You thus have an about one in two chance of not getting adequate sleep.** This is important for many reasons.

Sleep isn't a passive state of relaxation. Instead, **sleep is an active state of healing**. The sleeping brain is busy clearing accumulated neurotransmitters, heavy molecules, and other gunk. Your endocrine glands are being regulated and your body and mind get an opportunity to recover. Sleep-wake cycle is intimately related to other circadian rhythms such as the blood pressure, body temperature, and cortisol. Disruption of this cycle increases risk of heart disease, diabetes, cancer, and can predispose to early death.[25]

> Sleep isn't a state of passive relaxation. Sleep is an active state of healing.

Parallel with the other phenomena, the number of circulating immune cells also oscillates during the day,[26] as does their activity as manifested for example by the cytokine production. **Insufficient sleep increases susceptibility to viral infections,[27] decreases antibody response to vaccination,[28] and predisposes to inflammation**, partly by influencing cytokine secretion.[29,30] Lack of sleep increases circulating neutrophils,[31,32] and impairs NK cell activity.[32] NK cells are extremely important in your fight against the viruses.

Suggested actions:

Here are three ideas to improve your sleep:
- **Remove barriers**
- **Commit to a discipline**
- **Consider seeing a sleep specialist**

Remove barriers: Create a peaceful atmosphere in your bedroom. Keep the lighting dim, avoid flashy screens (TV, Smartphones, Tablets) as much as possible, lower the noise, and surround yourself with images and messages calm your mind. Avoid taking stimulants late in the day. Bypass eating heavy meals or doing vigorous exercise a few hours prior to sleeping. Also minimize (to the extent you can) visiting worries or emotionally taxing thoughts late during the day.

Commit to a discipline: Commit to a predictable sleeping and waking up time, while being more thoughtful about the daytime naps since they can sometimes interfere with the night-time sleep. Maintaining a sleep diary can help with this process.

Consider seeing a sleep specialist: If your partner has noticed you snore at night, if you wake up tired or with a headache, if you get drowsy during the day or behind the wheel, then it will be good to consult your primary healthcare provider and perhaps your sleep specialist. With poor sleep or with sleep apnea, you may be limiting oxygen supply to your brain for a large part of the night. That can't be healthy and deserves your full attention.

A brain that hasn't slept well functions like a physiologically older brain. **The immune system of a person who doesn't sleep well starts behaving like that of someone ten years older than him or her.** Such an immune system predisposes you to infection.

Perhaps the greatest barrier to your sleep is the tremendous backlog of work. You feel your sleeping time is a non-productive time. That's a common but

> Count sleep in your productive time.

unhelpful perspective. **No one will credit you if because of immune suppression and inflammation from lack of sleep, you catch a serious infection, develop a metabolic condition, or total your car.**

Remember—To be awake is human, to sleep is divine!

4. Build Physical Vitality

Our physical bodies from the outside look like two identical halves that are glued in the middle. Why do we have two lungs, two kidneys, and such a long intestine and colon? One reason is to create a reserve.

People who donate their one kidney live a normal life. Removing large parts of the liver and intestine doesn't change life expectancy. My father has spent sixty good years with one functioning eye. My friend has won multiple marathon races working with one lung.

The purpose of building physical vitality is two-fold:
- **Empower the immune system, and**
- **Build physical reserve in case an illness takes out part of an organ**

Two important questions

Can exercise help my immune system?
Am I optimally active during the day?

The science:

A large number of studies have evaluated the effect of exercise on your immune system. After a good review of the literature, my bottom-line conclusion is this: **Moderate physical activity (compared to sedentary lifestyle) improves immunity and protects from infections.**

Mind the word moderate here. If you start running marathons every week, you could tax your body and hurt your immune system (both innate and adaptive),[33] although this contention has been recently challenged in research.

> Moderate physical activity is better than sedentary lifestyle and also very vigorous physical activity.

Moderate exercise on the other hand can enhance immune response to vaccination (to flu and pneumonia vaccinations), reduce inflammation, and improve immune surveillance.[34] Overall **when it comes to the immune system, perhaps 30 minutes a day is better than three hours**.[35]

Exercise decreases inflammation by decreasing stress hormones and inflammatory cytokine levels in the blood.[36] Exercise also decreases percentage of body fat and macrophages in the fatty tissue, activates the cholinergic anti-inflammatory pathway, among other mechanisms.[37]

The effect of exercise on vaccination is particularly helpful for groups that are less likely to have a robust response to vaccination.[38,39]

While we have the most information about aerobic exercise, resistance training is also helpful for decreasing inflammatory markers particularly when added to the aerobic exercise.[40,41]

An important subset where exercise is particularly important is among the seniors. Regular exercise lowers inflammatory cytokines, enhances adaptive immunity, improves NK cell activity and lowers the number of senescent T cells.[42] While exercise may not completely reverse the effect of old age on the immune system, research is fairly compelling pointing to its considerable benefit.

Suggested actions:

Three suggested actions to benefit from exercise are:

- **Do something, however little**
- **Remain agile**
- **Build some muscles**

Do something, however little: You do not have to get into a vigorous regimen to get immune benefits from the exercise. Instead, start with something small and build from there. An important benefit of doing something is that it will increase your perception of wellbeing, that by itself can enhance your health. Keep in mind that if you have been sedentary for a

> Perception of wellbeing by itself can improve your health.

long time, it will help to talk to your healthcare provider to make sure you do not need any baseline testing before starting the exercise program.

Remain agile: Equally important to focused aerobic activity is to remain agile during the day. Some researchers call it NEAT (Non-exercise activity thermogenesis). Interesting research shows that NEAT can be an important source of weight management.[43] Further, convincing research shows that prolonged sitting (several hours at a time during the day) can increase your risk of diabetes, heart disease, stroke, cancer, and early death. Breaking your sitting time with intermittent walking can minimize these risks.[44,45]

Build some muscles: With research supporting the benefit of resistance exercise, invest a few minutes during the day to increase your muscle mass. It can simply be doing a few pushups, walking up and down the stairs, lifting some weights, or more. It might help to talk to a fitness expert to help customize the program to your strength and needs.

Practice Yoga or Tai Chi

While Yoga and Tai Chi teachers might see these practices as more about balance and mental and spiritual growth, both **Yoga and Tai Chi also involve considerable physical activity and definitely help your immune system.**

For example, a review of 16 studies showed that Tai Chi improves cell mediated immunity and the antibody response following vaccination.[46] Similarly, Tai Chi improved T cell function in patients with diabetes,[47] and improved varicella-zoster specific immunity among seniors.[48]

> Practice Yoga and Tai Chi, not just for emotional and physical benefits, but also to improve your immune system.

Similarly, a review of 15 studies suggested that a steady practice of yoga can lower inflammatory markers (including IL-6 and TNF-alpha) and might enhance adaptive and mucosal immunity.[49] A more recent study among patients with depression confirmed these findings.[50] Yoga also improves high blood pressure, diabetes, and multiple musculoskeletal conditions.[51]

If you have considered giving Yoga or Tai Chi a try, now may be a perfect time, to help your immune system. Both Yoga and Tai Chi also have a powerful effect on calming your mind. That's where we are going next.

5. Calm Your Mind

Stress is your struggle with what is, what was, or what might be.
When stressed you are in a state of war—with the world and with yourself.

> ## Two important questions
>
> Does stress hurt my immune system?
> How do I lower my stress?

The science

As a society, we are experiencing very high stress, from the excessive cognitive and emotional load most of us have to carry each day. Further, the world keeps producing novel threats for which we are little prepared. The element of surprise and unpredictability is tremendously unnerving.[52]

> Many of us experience high levels of stress because of excessive cognitive and emotional load.

The resulting fear epidemic hurts us in two ways. It decreases your immune system's ability to fight the infection (for example, by decreasing NK cell activity).[53] Fear (and other negative emotions) also increase the risk of unhealthy inflammation.[54] For many infections, an exaggerated immune response with its attendant inflammation can hurt as much as the infection itself.

Stress weakens your immune response by impairing dendritic cell function,[55] decreasing NK cell activity,[56] and lowering antibody production.[57-59] Stress thus hurts all the different arms of the immune system.[60] Stress also predisposes to inflammation.[61]

No demographic and no infection are protected from the effect of stress. The elderly who are stressed have lower response to the flu vaccine.[62] Workers with high effort-reward imbalance and overcommitment have lower immunity.[63] Stressed people experience higher risk of bacterial as well as viral infections such as herpes flare up.[64]

Similar to stress, both depression and anxiety hurt both innate and adaptive immunity,[65] and predispose to inflammation.[66,67] **Further, inflammation by itself may predispose to depression, trapping us in a feedback loop.**[68]

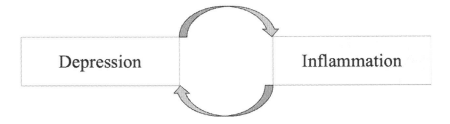

Importantly, **decreasing stress can reverse several of the immune changes associated with stress.**[69,70] Also, maintaining a positive outlook through a stressful situation can limit the adverse inflammatory effect of the stressor.[71]

Suggested actions

Stress management is an extensive topic that can take us in many different directions. I will present here three simple strategies that might be of value.

- **Eliminate optional stressors**
- **Boost your resilience**
- **Practice meditation**

Eliminate optional stressors: Pick at least one of the following that might be increasing your stress:

- Too much time with the news
- Taking negative people at their face value
- Letting others who don't care much about you, influence your self-worth
- Setting unrealistic expectations of yourself
- Wanting to please everyone

To the extent you can, change one of the stressors mentioned above. **Cut down your dose of daily news, give the negative people an eviction notice from your brain's real estate, believe in those who believe in you, set realistic expectations of yourself softening your instinct of perfectionism, and let go of the desire to please everyone.**

> Many of the stress management approaches converge to practicing self-kindness.

Many of these suggestions converge to one simple idea: be kind to yourself (self-compassion). **Greater your self-compassion, better your sleep, immunity, and overall physical health**.[72] Interesting research shows that for people exposed to a stressor, a better sense of self is associated with lower inflammatory response.[73]

Boost your resilience: Resilience is the core strength you use to lift the load of life. Resilience is your ability to withstand adversity, bounce back from adversity, and grow despite life's downturns. My team has developed some very specific resilience practices such as the morning gratitude, the two-minute rule, curious moments, kind attention, and resilient mindset. **Develop greater resilience by inviting five timeless principles into your life: gratitude, compassion,**

> The five principles that can help you become more resilient are gratitude, compassion, acceptance, meaning, and forgiveness.

acceptance, meaning, and forgiveness. Consider visiting resilientoption.com for more information.

Practice meditation: Most meditation types help the immune system. The most studied among meditations is the mindfulness meditation. Mindfulness meditation enhances NK cell activity, lowers inflammatory molecules,[74] helps with neurogenic inflammation,[75] and enhances antibody response to vaccination.[76,77] Similar beneficial results have been seen with other meditation programs, a broad spectrum of mind-body approaches,[78] and relaxation.[79-81] Interestingly some of these changes correlate with increased left prefrontal cortex activity, that in turn is associated with experiencing positive emotions.[82]

Meditation is one skill that is easy to learn but difficult to master. Keep measured expectations and start with a very simple practice. Just as you can't swim like a dolphin in a few weeks, you won't experience uninterrupted calm with a few weeks of meditation.

You can pick one of the simple meditations developed by my team that are available online. They include *Calm and Energize*, *Rhythm*, and

Morning Gratitude, all available on YouTube. Several excellent vendors offer well-thought-out meditation programs.

In addition to meditation, you can use other mind-body approaches such as guided imagery or hypnosis.[83,84] Pick a practice that is easy, accessible, aligns with your worldview, and connects you with others —the next step in our journey together.

6. Feel Connected

We experience most of our life in three relationships—with the self, with others, and with what we consider sacred. Optimal integration of these three relationships is a recipe for a content life. Presently, I will focus on the latter two.

Nurture deeper relationships

Two important questions
How relationships affect the immune system? Am I satisfied with my relationships?

The science

Relationships touch us deeper than the skin. For example, perceived loneliness doesn't just make us sad. **Loneliness is associated with upregulation of the genes that predispose to inflammation and downregulation of the genes that produce a good immune response.**[85-87] Lonely people thus have higher level of inflammatory markers and show a greater inflammatory response to a social challenge.[88]

Adversarial connections have similar effects as loneliness.[89] Thus, people with adversarial connections experience higher inflammation which may by itself negatively affect mood.[90] Further, the greater the inflammation, the higher the social sensitivity, putting people in a downward spiral leading to increasing loneliness.[91] Several pathways connect social support to immune system including the brain, the endocrine system, emotional stress response, and health behaviors.[92]

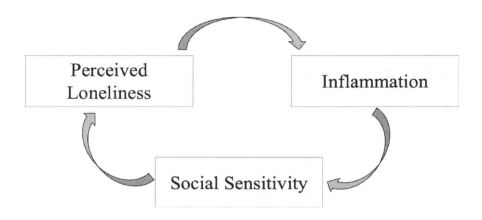

Social support on the other hand is associated with lower inflammation,[93] better immune response,[94] and is thus intimately related to your health.[95] Social support also enhances immune response to vaccination.[96] Further, **social support is associated with stronger innate antiviral immunity,[91] which is very important when we face threats for which we do not have good vaccines or drugs.[97]**

The more connected you feel with others, the better your immune system.

In the elderly, social support is associated with healthier immune system.[98] The spouses of patients with cancer had more robust NK cell activity if they perceived good social support.[99] In patients with HIV, a low perception of attachment was associated with a much more rapid decline in the CD4 cell count.[100]

In the context of social connections, two areas of particular interest are anger control and kindness. Interesting research shows that **poor anger control slows healing**.[101] **Even memory of anger triggering event can increase production of inflammatory chemicals** (TNF alpha and IL-6 production).[102]

Importantly, **hostile marital interactions increase inflammatory response, markedly slowing healing,**[103] and are associated with higher sympathetic activity.[104] **Better relationship among couples on the other hand leads to better health outcomes**.[105]

Kindness is associated with lower inflammatory gene expression.[106] Self-kindness has wide ranging positive effects on physical health.[72] Similarly, forgiveness, that often emerges from practicing kindness, improves T helper cells, an important part of healthy immune system.[107]

> Kindness not only calms your mind, but also calms your body's inflammation.

With all this science to support the value of our relationships, let's next put one or two ideas into practice.

Suggested actions:

Three suggested actions you can take to improve your immunity through connections are:

- **Do something nice**
- **Be good to your neighbors**
- **Forgive**

Do something nice: Make a list of the people closest to you. For the next one week every single day, plan one nice thing for at least one person in this list. It could be an expression of gratitude, buying a surprise small gift, making an uplifting phone call, giving undivided attention, or something else. Such an action will help both of you generate a healthier immune response.

Be good to your neighbors: Your neighbors have outsized effect on your wellbeing, almost as strong if not stronger than your loved ones. Invest some time thinking about how you can enhance your connection with them. Engage in conversation, express gratitude, shower authentic praise, and look out for each other's wellbeing.

> Your relationship with neighbors has a powerful effect on your wellbeing.

Forgive: Global concerns and crises are times to remember what is most important. **This isn't a time to fear; it is a time to forgive.** Remember that forgiveness is for you not for the other person. **By forgiving, you free your brain's real estate from the other person.** You are improving your health, connections, and choosing to live by your values. You do not have to tell them you have forgiven them.

Think of someone who has hurt you in the past. One of the best ways you can enhance your immune system is by choosing to forgive that person.

As you commit investing your time and energy to relationships, keep in mind that the greatest impact of relationships is through real life friends and not social media.[108] This is partly because the quality of social connections is more important than quantity.[109] Let a thousand likes on social media not be an excuse to stop hugging your mom.

Invest Time in Spirituality

Before concluding this chapter, I wish to provide a gentle reminder that **the practice of spirituality does wonders to your immune system.**

Spiritual practices enhance immunity by influencing the number and subset of immune cells (helper and cytotoxic T cells).[110] A large study analyzing multiple previous studies showed that religiosity and spirituality are correlated with lower levels of inflammatory markers.[111] Further, even more inspiring, **a review of 21 studies showed enhancing spirituality improves several immune parameters**.[112]

Spirituality helps through many different mechanisms. They include deeper social connections, lower stress, better health behaviors, and likely a direct effect. Although we need to continue researching the benefits of spirituality, I have no doubt that inclusive spiritual practices will help your immune system and your health.[113] Given that 70 percent of the people consider religion/spirituality as an important part of their life, this is a very important way to enhance physical health.

Invest a little time in a practice you love. It will help your physical body as well as make you happier, which is our next step in this journey together.

7. Be A Little Happier

Happiness is experiencing a preponderance of positive emotions. Authentic happiness is deep sustained fulfillment that you get from living a good, virtuous, and meaningful life. To that, you can also add having some fun!

Broadly, happiness has three sources: *life satisfaction* from feeling content, *pleasure* related to a delightful experience, and *joy* related to pursuing and fulfilling an inspiring meaning.

Two important questions

Can happiness help my health?
How can I get happier?

The science

Happiness doesn't just feel good. When you are happier, you are more likely to –

- speak positive words
- help others
- forgive
- feel grateful and express gratitude
- be healthier
- live longer

Happiness enhances health and longevity[114] by improving genetic expression,[115] enhancing immunity and autonomic balance, decreasing inflammatory markers,[116] improving lifestyle, and enhancing social connections.[117]

Further, your happiness is infectious. **When you feel happy (and show it), people close to you not only become more joyous, they also become physically healthier.**

Laughter, a physical expression of happiness, is a broad-spectrum health enhancing activity. Laughing upregulates your NK cell immune response genes,[118,119] and decreases pro-inflammatory cytokines, particularly in people with inflammatory state.[120] **Watching a funny video can increase NK cell activity for as long as 12 hours.**[121] Angry or anxious response to a social situation does the opposite, increasing your inflammation.[122]

> A good laugh can improve your immunity for as long as 12 hours.

It takes 43 muscles to frown and only 17 to smile. Smile and laugh to help your health and immunity.

An important ingredient of happiness is hope. **Hope protects you from the inflammatory and immune suppressing effects of stress**.[123] Optimism is also associated with higher NK cell activity, improving your anti-viral response.[124,125] In addition to the immune system, optimism has wide ranging positive effects on almost every health outcome studied.[126] The effect of optimism on the immune system is central to its beneficial effect on overall wellbeing.[127]

Music is another simple yet powerful source of happiness.[128] Research shows that **the predictable harmful effect of stress on immune and**

inflammatory markers can be reversed by music.[129] These benefits have also been seen in the seniors.[130]

Music in a social context is especially beneficial. Choir singing is associated with improvement in immune markers.[131] Drumming over a period of 10 weeks is associated with a shift from pro-inflammatory toward an anti-inflammatory immune state.[132] Drumming is also reported to enhance NK cell activity.[133]

> Music and massage are simple and powerful approaches to increase happiness and improve immune response.

If you wish to pamper yourself, consider also massage! Aromatherapy massage lowers stress and inflammatory immune markers.[134] A review of five studies suggested that massage improved immunological recovery after intense exercise.[135] Massage improved NK cell activity,[136] and decreased CD4 cell decline in patients with HIV.[135] Even a single session of massage can improve physiological markers that are associated with better immunity and inflammation.[137]

Suggested actions:

Here are three approaches to enhance happiness. Remember that *feeling loved at home* and *respected at work* are the key to lasting happiness.[138]

- **Pick one idea**
- **Get a massage**
- **Invite music**

Pick one idea: Here is a list of some of the ideas to enhance happiness (a few are repeated from above)

- Become physically active
- Eat healthy

- Cultivate real-life friends
- Pamper yourself (at least occasionally)
- Feel grateful
- Lower expectations
- Create a "Not to do" list
- Live each day with purpose
- Help others
- Do interesting projects
- Be kind to others
- Be kind to yourself
- Nurture hope
- Forgive
- Count your blessings
- Practice spirituality

As you implement these ideas remember that an analysis of 1.5 million words showed that **we speak happier words when we talk about the good people in our life compared to reference to material things.**[139] Hence, **one of the easiest and most effective path to finding enduring happiness is through relationships**.

> Focusing on positive relationships makes us happier than focusing on material things.

Get a massage: If you feel upto it, consider getting a massage to help enhance your wellbeing. This can be massage by a professional or self-massage.

Add music to life: Music has powerful influence on our wellbeing. You can keep a committed time listening to music, add music as a background to anything else you are doing, and also participate in group activities that bring music to your life such as choir, drumming, and more.

As you implement happiness-promoting activities, keep in mind that **happiness doesn't mean suppressing all negative emotions**. **The happiest people are those who allow themselves to experience authentic emotions, instead of bottling up negative emotions.** Further, research showed that people who allowed themselves to cry experienced an improvement in inflammatory markers.[140] Thus, **be emotionally authentic, instead of forcing positivity.**

In whatever you do, be kind to yourself.

8. Choose the Right Chemicals

Many of the approaches I have outlined above act through changing your body's chemical milieu. Eliminating harmful chemicals from your body and adding useful chemicals is an excellent direct strategy to enhance your immunity.

Say Bye to Harmful Chemicals

> ### Two important questions
>
> Am I taking any harmful chemical?
> How can I get rid of this harmful chemical?

The science

Your body can receive harmful chemicals through eating, drinking, inhaling, or other means. The three most harmful chemicals are smoking, excessive alcohol, and drugs of abuse.

Cigarette smoking has severe and widespread damaging effect on both innate and adaptive immunity. Thus, smoking affects T helper cells, regulatory T cells, CD8+ T cells, B cells, macrophages, and NK cells.[1] Smoking also impairs immune response to vaccination,[141] and switches the immune response to a more inflammatory one.[142]

Similarly, excessive alcohol intake predisposes to inflammatory immune changes.[143] While mild to moderate alcohol intake may help the immune system, heavy intake hurts the functioning of T and B cells, predisposing to infections.[144,145]

Combined smoking and excessive alcohol use have a remarkably harmful effect on the immune system combined with increasing predisposition to inflammation.[143] These changes increase your risk of pneumonia and other infections. Further, a review of 20 studies showed that smoking increases the risk of hospital and ICU admissions in patients with the flu.[146]

> Smoking and excessive alcohol intake hurt our immunity, cause inflammation, and increase the risk of infections.

Like smoking and excessive alcohol use, almost every single drug of abuse has been associated with impairment of the immune system with or without predisposition to inflammation.

In addition, think about the chemicals you might be ingesting through your food (excessive preservatives, colors, pesticides, heavy metals, bacteria, and more), water (heavy metals such as lead, bacteria, and more) in the air (pollution, radon, fuel exhausts, and more), and through the skin (cosmetic products in particular). While we do not need to be paranoid about every little chemical, **taking a few prudent steps to minimize the load of immune altering chemicals will help your overall health, particularly your immune system.**

Suggested actions:

Here are three approaches to decrease the load of chemicals on your body:

- **Stop smoking**

- **Decrease alcohol intake**
- **Decrease other harmful chemicals**

Stop smoking: If you smoke cigarettes or consume tobacco in another form, take the necessary steps to quit this habit. It is extremely important for your overall health and the health of your immune system. Everything else being equal, your chances of a more severe infection are much higher with smoking. Access the CDC tobacco quit line, call 1-800-QUIT-NOW, or contact your health care provider for the next step.

Decrease alcohol intake: Mild to moderate alcohol intake may help the immunity, while heavy alcohol intake (binge drinking 5 or more days in the past month) harms every aspect of your life. If you are a heavy drinker consider accessing SAMHSA's helpline at 1-800-662-HELP (4357) or contact your healthcare team. SAMSHA stands for Substance Abuse and Mental Health Services Administration. You can access the same resources for quitting other substances.

Decrease other harmful chemicals: Take a stock of the food you eat, the water you drink, and the air you breathe. Without becoming obsessive compulsive and paranoid, take a rational approach toward decreasing the dose of harmful chemicals that enter your body.

Say Hello to Helpful Compounds

Two important questions
Do supplements affect the immune system? Should I start taking any supplements?

The science

The best source of helpful compounds are the ones packed by nature—as fruits and vegetables. But in some situations, specific supplements are helpful. For example, patients with malabsorption need supplementation with vitamins and minerals, elderly with low B12 absorption will be helped by extra B12 intake, people on vegan low-calorie diet may be helped by a multi-vitamin and mineral supplement, people living in the northern hemisphere with limited sun exposure might be helped by extra vitamin D.

Here are a few interesting findings from research studies about the effect of supplements or their deficiency on the immune system:

Vitamin A and D: These two vitamins influence lymphocyte activation and division, T-helper-cell differentiation, tissue-specific lymphocyte homing, the production of specific antibody isotypes, and regulation of the immune response.[147]

Blueberries and grapes: Two compounds in these fruits, resveratrol and pterostilbene enhance immune function.[148]

Bovine colostrum: Bovine colostrum enhances NK cell activity and enhances immune response to RSV and the influenza virus.[149,150] In a study, use of bovine colostrum was associated with lower number of days with upper respiratory illness.[151]

Broccoli: The phytochemicals in Brassica vegetables of which Broccoli is one, help stimulate the immune system.[152]

Vitamin C: Vitamin C improves NK cell activity, lymphocyte proliferation, and activity of the immune cells. Optimal intake of vitamin C is helpful, but mega doses are of dubious benefit.[153] Further, when you ingest very high doses of vitamin C or another compound, you overwhelm your body's metabolic pathways. That can harm you in the short and the long term.

Echinacea: Echinacea has both immunomodulatory and anti-inflammatory effect. In a review of six studies, Echinacea can lower the risk of recurrent respiratory tract infections and complications from these infections.[154]

Vitamin E: Vitamin E influences NK cells, macrophages, T cell, and B cell function.[155] Vitamin E supplementation can improve cell-mediated immunity, oxidative stress,[156] and enhances immune response in the elderly.[157]

Garlic: Garlic can enhance the function of NK cells, lymphocytes, and macrophages, and modulate production of inflammatory molecules and immunoglobulins.[158,159] Garlic supplementation might decrease the severity,[160] as well as the incidence of cold and flu.[161]

Ginger: Ginger has excellent anti-inflammatory properties and might be useful as a component of a healthy diet that supports the immune system.[162]

Micronutrients: We were introduced to micronutrients in chapter 3. They are important in the smooth functioning of the immune system.[163]

Probiotics: Many different probiotics are immune modulators and decrease the inflammatory response.[164] Some of the beneficial effects of probiotics may be through modifying the gut flora.[165] Probiotics also enhance NK cell activity.[166]

Turmeric: Turmeric has broad ranging effects on the immune system including T and B lymphocytes, macrophages, and NK cells.[167] Curcumin, the active compound in turmeric has a particularly important role in limiting inflammation.[168]

The above is only a partial list, with many more supplements such as different types of mushrooms, ginseng, green tea, and others known to have anti-inflammatory and immune enhancing effects. In general, many of these supplements have intriguing effect on the immune cells but their benefit on the risks and outcomes of an infection have not been fully studied

> Many supplements have shown immune enhancing and anti-inflammatory properties.

Presently, it is difficult to recommend one particular supplement for its immune benefits. A good approach might be to add blueberries, grapes, broccoli, garlic, ginger, probiotics, and turmeric as part of a healthy diet, and correct any micronutrient deficiency.

9. Build Your Immune Resilience: A Three-Month Program

In chapters 3-8, I have provided a review of some of the research related to different approaches to help your immune system. As you can see, there is a lot you can do to prepare your body and mind to better face today's challenge and all future threats. Further, when you move from passivity and fear to taking control, that by itself empowers your physical body and the immune system. I invite you to make that transition.

Let's put it all together in two simple steps so you can implement a few useful changes in the coming days and weeks.

Step 1: Look at the 15 activities below. Rank them in your order of priority based on their importance and how feasible it is to take the next step.

Immune Resilience Activity	My Priority Rank (#1 to #15)	Next Step
Correct micronutrient deficiency		Refer to chapter 3
Get adequate sleep		Refer to chapter 3
Do moderate physical activity		Refer to chapter 4
Manage my stress better		Refer to chapter 5
Build emotional resilience		Refer to chapter 5

Practice meditation or another mind-body practice		Refer to chapter 5
Feel socially connected / Improve relationships		Refer to chapter 6
Invest time in a personally meaningful spiritual practice		Refer to chapter 6
Nurture hope		Refer to chapter 7
Laugh more		Refer to chapter 7
Get a massage		Refer to chapter 7
Add music to my life		Refer to chapter 7
Stop smoking		Refer to chapter 8
Decrease alcohol intake		Refer to chapter 8
Consider taking a supplement		Refer to chapter 8

Step 2: Build the following table based on your order of priority and populate the best next step. Implement the change over a week (or faster or slower, whatever works for you), and incrementally add more activities. Build this table one activity at a time.

My Priority Rank	My Immune Resilience Activity	My Planned Next Step
1		
2		
3		
4		
5		
6		
7		
8		
9		
10		
11		
12		
13		
14		
15		

I hope you feel empowered with the science and ideas I have shared above.

Let's respond to the challenge we all face today by becoming stronger, wiser, kinder, and better connected with each other. Implement changes that make you physically, emotionally, and immunologically resilient. If we do that, I strongly believe we will have the last laugh not the microscopic pathogen/s that don't mean us well. We will also be better prepared for any future challenge.

Let's convert this moment of disruption into a moment of transformation.

My warmest wishes and deepest prayers for your and your family's health and wellbeing.

Take good care of yourself. You are precious.

- Amit

References

1. Qiu F, Liang CL, Liu H, et al. Impacts of cigarette smoking on immune responsiveness: Up and down or upside down? Oncotarget 2017;8:268-84.
2. Jones DS, Podolsky SH, Greene JA. The burden of disease and the changing task of medicine. The New England journal of medicine 2012;366:2333-8.
3. Gates B. Responding to Covid-19 - A Once-in-a-Century Pandemic? The New England journal of medicine 2020.
4. Murray JF. A century of tuberculosis. American journal of respiratory and critical care medicine 2004;169:1181-6.
5. Brydon L, Walker C, Wawrzyniak A, et al. Synergistic effects of psychological and immune stressors on inflammatory cytokine and sickness responses in humans. Brain, behavior, and immunity 2009;23:217-24.
6. Cunningham-Rundles S, McNeeley DF, Moon A. Mechanisms of nutrient modulation of the immune response. The Journal of allergy and clinical immunology 2005;115:1119-28; quiz 29.
7. Maggini S, Wintergerst ES, Beveridge S, Hornig DH. Selected vitamins and trace elements support immune function by strengthening epithelial barriers and cellular and humoral immune responses. The British journal of nutrition 2007;98 Suppl 1:S29-35.
8. Wintergerst ES, Maggini S, Hornig DH. Contribution of selected vitamins and trace elements to immune function. Annals of nutrition & metabolism 2007;51:301-23.
9. Zheng L, Wang Q, Cheng X, et al. Perceived reputation of others modulates empathic neural responses. Experimental brain research 2016;234:125-32.
10. Chandra RK. Nutrition and the immune system: an introduction. The American journal of clinical nutrition 1997;66:460s-3s.
11. Gombart AF, Pierre A, Maggini S. A Review of Micronutrients and the Immune System-Working in Harmony to Reduce the Risk of Infection. Nutrients 2020;12.
12. Scheurig AC, Thorand B, Fischer B, Heier M, Koenig W. Association between the intake of vitamins and trace elements from supplements and C-reactive protein: results of the MONICA/KORA Augsburg study. European journal of clinical nutrition 2008;62:127-37.
13. Lumeng CN. Innate immune activation in obesity. Molecular aspects of medicine 2013;34:12-29.
14. Andersen CJ, Murphy KE, Fernandez ML. Impact of Obesity and Metabolic Syndrome on Immunity. Advances in nutrition (Bethesda, Md) 2016;7:66-75.
15. Milner JJ, Beck MA. The impact of obesity on the immune response to infection. The Proceedings of the Nutrition Society 2012;71:298-306.
16. Esfahani A, Wong JM, Truan J, et al. Health effects of mixed fruit and vegetable concentrates: a systematic review of the clinical interventions. Journal of the American College of Nutrition 2011;30:285-94.
17. Holt EM, Steffen LM, Moran A, et al. Fruit and vegetable consumption and its relation to markers of inflammation and oxidative stress in adolescents. Journal of the American Dietetic Association 2009;109:414-21.

18.   Nantz MP, Rowe CA, Nieves C, Jr., Percival SS. Immunity and antioxidant capacity in humans is enhanced by consumption of a dried, encapsulated fruit and vegetable juice concentrate. The Journal of nutrition 2006;136:2606-10.

19.   Lamprecht M, Oettl K, Schwaberger G, Hofmann P, Greilberger JF. Several indicators of oxidative stress, immunity, and illness improved in trained men consuming an encapsulated juice powder concentrate for 28 weeks. The Journal of nutrition 2007;137:2737-41.

20.   Yu R, Park JW, Kurata T, Erickson KL. Modulation of select immune responses by dietary capsaicin. International journal for vitamin and nutrition research Internationale Zeitschrift fur Vitamin- und Ernahrungsforschung Journal international de vitaminologie et de nutrition 1998;68:114-9.

21.   Shin HS, See HJ, Jung SY, et al. Turmeric (Curcuma longa) attenuates food allergy symptoms by regulating type 1/type 2 helper T cells (Th1/Th2) balance in a mouse model of food allergy. Journal of ethnopharmacology 2015;175:21-9.

22.   Turbitt WJ, Demark-Wahnefried W, Peterson CM, Norian LA. Targeting Glucose Metabolism to Enhance Immunotherapy: Emerging Evidence on Intermittent Fasting and Calorie Restriction Mimetics. Frontiers in immunology 2019;10:1402.

23.   Mindikoglu AL, Abdulsada MM, Jain A, et al. Intermittent fasting from dawn to sunset for 30 consecutive days is associated with anticancer proteomic signature and upregulates key regulatory proteins of glucose and lipid metabolism, circadian clock, DNA repair, cytoskeleton remodeling, immune system and cognitive function in healthy subjects. Journal of proteomics 2020:103645.

24.   Sleep and Sleep Disorders. CDC, 2020. (Accessed January 28, 2020, at https://www.cdc.gov/sleep/data_statistics.html.)

25.   Cappuccio FP, D'Elia L, Strazzullo P, Miller MA. Sleep duration and all-cause mortality: a systematic review and meta-analysis of prospective studies. Sleep 2010;33:585-92.

26.   Elmadjian F, Pincus G. A study of the diurnal variations in circulating lymphocytes in normal and psychotic subjects. The Journal of clinical endocrinology and metabolism 1946;6:287-94.

27.   Prather AA, Janicki-Deverts D, Hall MH, Cohen S. Behaviorally Assessed Sleep and Susceptibility to the Common Cold. Sleep 2015;38:1353-9.

28.   Prather AA, Hall M, Fury JM, et al. Sleep and antibody response to hepatitis B vaccination. Sleep 2012;35:1063-9.

29.   Richardson MR, Churilla JR. Sleep Duration and C-Reactive Protein in US Adults. Southern medical journal 2017;110:314-7.

30.   Mullington JM, Simpson NS, Meier-Ewert HK, Haack M. Sleep loss and inflammation. Best practice & research Clinical endocrinology & metabolism 2010;24:775-84.

31.   Ingram LA, Simpson RJ, Malone E, Florida-James GD. Sleep disruption and its effect on lymphocyte redeployment following an acute bout of exercise. Brain, behavior, and immunity 2015;47:100-8.

32.   Besedovsky L, Lange T, Haack M. The Sleep-Immune Crosstalk in Health and Disease. Physiological reviews 2019;99:1325-80.

33.   Simpson RJ, Kunz H, Agha N, Graff R. Exercise and the Regulation of Immune Functions. Progress in molecular biology and translational science 2015;135:355-80.

34. Nieman DC, Wentz LM. The compelling link between physical activity and the body's defense system. Journal of sport and health science 2019;8:201-17.

35. Dimitrov S, Hulteng E, Hong S. Inflammation and exercise: Inhibition of monocytic intracellular TNF production by acute exercise via beta2-adrenergic activation. Brain, behavior, and immunity 2017;61:60-8.

36. Ortega E. The "bioregulatory effect of exercise" on the innate/inflammatory responses. Journal of physiology and biochemistry 2016;72:361-9.

37. Woods JA, Vieira VJ, Keylock KT. Exercise, inflammation, and innate immunity. Immunology and allergy clinics of North America 2009;29:381-93.

38. Pascoe AR, Fiatarone Singh MA, Edwards KM. The effects of exercise on vaccination responses: a review of chronic and acute exercise interventions in humans. Brain, behavior, and immunity 2014;39:33-41.

39. Edwards KM, Booy R. Effects of exercise on vaccine-induced immune responses. Human vaccines & immunotherapeutics 2013;9:907-10.

40. Khosravi N, Stoner L, Farajivafa V, Hanson ED. Exercise training, circulating cytokine levels and immune function in cancer survivors: A meta-analysis. Brain, behavior, and immunity 2019;81:92-104.

41. Freidenreich DJ, Volek JS. Immune responses to resistance exercise. Exercise immunology review 2012;18:8-41.

42. Simpson RJ, Lowder TW, Spielmann G, Bigley AB, LaVoy EC, Kunz H. Exercise and the aging immune system. Ageing research reviews 2012;11:404-20.

43. Levine JA. Nonexercise activity thermogenesis--liberating the life-force. Journal of internal medicine 2007;262:273-87.

44. Larsson SC, Wolk A. Sedentary leisure-time in relation to mortality and survival time. Journal of science and medicine in sport 2019;22:562-7.

45. Cabanas-Sanchez V, Guallar-Castillon P, Higueras-Fresnillo S, Rodriguez-Artalejo F, Martinez-Gomez D. Changes in Sitting Time and Cardiovascular Mortality in Older Adults. American journal of preventive medicine 2018;54:419-22.

46. Ho RT, Wang CW, Ng SM, et al. The effect of t'ai chi exercise on immunity and infections: a systematic review of controlled trials. Journal of alternative and complementary medicine (New York, NY) 2013;19:389-96.

47. Yeh SH, Chuang H, Lin LW, et al. Regular Tai Chi Chuan exercise improves T cell helper function of patients with type 2 diabetes mellitus with an increase in T-bet transcription factor and IL-12 production. British journal of sports medicine 2009;43:845-50.

48. Irwin MR, Pike JL, Cole JC, Oxman MN. Effects of a behavioral intervention, Tai Chi Chih, on varicella-zoster virus specific immunity and health functioning in older adults. Psychosomatic medicine 2003;65:824-30.

49. Falkenberg RI, Eising C, Peters ML. Yoga and immune system functioning: a systematic review of randomized controlled trials. Journal of behavioral medicine 2018;41:467-82.

50. Nugent NR, Brick L, Armey MF, Tyrka AR, Ridout KK, Uebelacker LA. Benefits of Yoga on IL-6: Findings from a Randomized Controlled Trial of Yoga for Depression. Behavioral medicine (Washington, DC) 2019:1-10.

51. Chu P, Gotink RA, Yeh GY, Goldie SJ, Hunink MG. The effectiveness of yoga in modifying risk factors for cardiovascular disease and metabolic syndrome: A systematic

review and meta-analysis of randomized controlled trials. European journal of preventive cardiology 2016;23:291-307.

52.   Kelvin DJ, Rubino S. Fear of the novel coronavirus. Journal of infection in developing countries 2020;14:1-2.

53.   Segerstrom SC, Glover DA, Craske MG, Fahey JL. Worry affects the immune response to phobic fear. Brain, behavior, and immunity 1999;13:80-92.

54.   Graham-Engeland JE, Sin NL, Smyth JM, et al. Negative and positive affect as predictors of inflammation: Timing matters. Brain, behavior, and immunity 2018;74:222-30.

55.   Elftman MD, Hunzeker JT, Mellinger JC, Bonneau RH, Norbury CC, Truckenmiller ME. Stress-induced glucocorticoids at the earliest stages of herpes simplex virus-1 infection suppress subsequent antiviral immunity, implicating impaired dendritic cell function. Journal of immunology (Baltimore, Md : 1950) 2010;184:1867-75.

56.   Gerritsen W, Heijnen CJ, Wiegant VM, Bermond B, Frijda NH. Experimental social fear: immunological, hormonal, and autonomic concomitants. Psychosomatic medicine 1996;58:273-86.

57.   Pedersen AF, Zachariae R, Bovbjerg DH. Psychological stress and antibody response to influenza vaccination: a meta-analysis. Brain, behavior, and immunity 2009;23:427-33.

58.   Glaser R, Sheridan J, Malarkey WB, MacCallum RC, Kiecolt-Glaser JK. Chronic stress modulates the immune response to a pneumococcal pneumonia vaccine. Psychosomatic medicine 2000;62:804-7.

59.   Burns VE, Carroll D, Ring C, Drayson M. Antibody response to vaccination and psychosocial stress in humans: relationships and mechanisms. Vaccine 2003;21:2523-34.

60.   Segerstrom SC, Miller GE. Psychological stress and the human immune system: a meta-analytic study of 30 years of inquiry. Psychological bulletin 2004;130:601-30.

61.   Kiecolt-Glaser JK, Preacher KJ, MacCallum RC, Atkinson C, Malarkey WB, Glaser R. Chronic stress and age-related increases in the proinflammatory cytokine IL-6. Proceedings of the National Academy of Sciences of the United States of America 2003;100:9090-5.

62.   Kiecolt-Glaser JK, Glaser R, Gravenstein S, Malarkey WB, Sheridan J. Chronic stress alters the immune response to influenza virus vaccine in older adults. Proceedings of the National Academy of Sciences of the United States of America 1996;93:3043-7.

63.   Eddy P, Heckenberg R, Wertheim EH, Kent S, Wright BJ. A systematic review and meta-analysis of the effort-reward imbalance model of workplace stress with indicators of immune function. Journal of psychosomatic research 2016;91:1-8.

64.   Glaser R, Kiecolt-Glaser JK. Chronic stress modulates the virus-specific immune response to latent herpes simplex virus type 1. Annals of behavioral medicine : a publication of the Society of Behavioral Medicine 1997;19:78-82.

65.   Goyal S, Srivastava K, Kodange C, Bhat PS. Immunological changes in depression. Industrial psychiatry journal 2017;26:201-6.

66.   Vogelzangs N, de Jonge P, Smit JH, Bahn S, Penninx BW. Cytokine production capacity in depression and anxiety. Translational psychiatry 2016;6:e825.

67.   Jeenger J, Sharma M, Mathur DM, Amandeep. Associations of number and severity of depressive episodes with C-reactive protein and Interleukin-6. Asian journal of psychiatry 2017;27:71-5.

68.   Irwin MR, Cole S, Olmstead R, et al. Moderators for depressed mood and systemic and transcriptional inflammatory responses: a randomized controlled trial of endotoxin. Neuropsychopharmacology : official publication of the American College of Neuropsychopharmacology 2019;44:635-41.

69.   Abrahao CA, Bomfim E, Lopes-Junior LC, Pereira-da-Silva G. Complementary Therapies as a Strategy to Reduce Stress and Stimulate Immunity of Women With Breast Cancer. Journal of evidence-based integrative medicine 2019;24:2515690x19834169.

70.   Antoni MH, Dhabhar FS. The impact of psychosocial stress and stress management on immune responses in patients with cancer. Cancer 2019;125:1417-31.

71.   Aschbacher K, Epel E, Wolkowitz OM, Prather AA, Puterman E, Dhabhar FS. Maintenance of a positive outlook during acute stress protects against pro-inflammatory reactivity and future depressive symptoms. Brain, behavior, and immunity 2012;26:346-52.

72.   Phillips WJ, Hine DW. Self-compassion, physical health, and health behaviour: a meta-analysis. Health psychology review 2019:1-27.

73.   O'Donnell K, Brydon L, Wright CE, Steptoe A. Self-esteem levels and cardiovascular and inflammatory responses to acute stress. Brain, behavior, and immunity 2008;22:1241-7.

74.   Witek Janusek L, Tell D, Mathews HL. Mindfulness based stress reduction provides psychological benefit and restores immune function of women newly diagnosed with breast cancer: A randomized trial with active control. Brain, behavior, and immunity 2019;80:358-73.

75.   Rosenkranz MA, Lutz A, Perlman DM, et al. Reduced stress and inflammatory responsiveness in experienced meditators compared to a matched healthy control group. Psychoneuroendocrinology 2016;68:117-25.

76.   Heckenberg RA, Eddy P, Kent S, Wright BJ. Do workplace-based mindfulness meditation programs improve physiological indices of stress? A systematic review and meta-analysis. Journal of psychosomatic research 2018;114:62-71.

77.   Black DS, Slavich GM. Mindfulness meditation and the immune system: a systematic review of randomized controlled trials. Annals of the New York Academy of Sciences 2016;1373:13-24.

78.   Morgan N, Irwin MR, Chung M, Wang C. The effects of mind-body therapies on the immune system: meta-analysis. PloS one 2014;9:e100903.

79.   Keresztes M, Rudisch T, Tajti J, Ocsovszki I, Gardi J. Granulocyte activation in humans is modulated by psychological stress and relaxation. Stress (Amsterdam, Netherlands) 2007;10:271-81.

80.   Gruzelier JH. A review of the impact of hypnosis, relaxation, guided imagery and individual differences on aspects of immunity and health. Stress (Amsterdam, Netherlands) 2002;5:147-63.

81.   Gruzelier JH. The role of psychological intervention in modulating aspects of immune function in relation to health and well-being. International review of neurobiology 2002;52:383-417.

82.   Davidson RJ, Kabat-Zinn J, Schumacher J, et al. Alterations in brain and immune function produced by mindfulness meditation. Psychosomatic medicine 2003;65:564-70.
83.   Trakhtenberg EC. The effects of guided imagery on the immune system: a critical review. The International journal of neuroscience 2008;118:839-55.
84.   Bakke AC, Purtzer MZ, Newton P. The effect of hypnotic-guided imagery on psychological well-being and immune function in patients with prior breast cancer. Journal of psychosomatic research 2002;53:1131-7.
85.   Powell ND, Sloan EK, Bailey MT, et al. Social stress up-regulates inflammatory gene expression in the leukocyte transcriptome via beta-adrenergic induction of myelopoiesis. Proceedings of the National Academy of Sciences of the United States of America 2013;110:16574-9.
86.   Cole SW, Conti G, Arevalo JM, Ruggiero AM, Heckman JJ, Suomi SJ. Transcriptional modulation of the developing immune system by early life social adversity. Proceedings of the National Academy of Sciences of the United States of America 2012;109:20578-83.
87.   Cole SW, Capitanio JP, Chun K, Arevalo JM, Ma J, Cacioppo JT. Myeloid differentiation architecture of leukocyte transcriptome dynamics in perceived social isolation. Proceedings of the National Academy of Sciences of the United States of America 2015;112:15142-7.
88.   Eisenberger NI, Moieni M, Inagaki TK, Muscatell KA, Irwin MR. In Sickness and in Health: The Co-Regulation of Inflammation and Social Behavior. Neuropsychopharmacology : official publication of the American College of Neuropsychopharmacology 2017;42:242-53.
89.   Kiecolt-Glaser JK. Marriage, divorce, and the immune system. The American psychologist 2018;73:1098-108.
90.   Slavich GM, Irwin MR. From stress to inflammation and major depressive disorder: a social signal transduction theory of depression. Psychological bulletin 2014;140:774-815.
91.   Leschak CJ, Eisenberger NI. Two Distinct Immune Pathways Linking Social Relationships With Health: Inflammatory and Antiviral Processes. Psychosomatic medicine 2019;81:711-9.
92.   Kiecolt-Glaser JK, Gouin JP, Hantsoo L. Close relationships, inflammation, and health. Neuroscience and biobehavioral reviews 2010;35:33-8.
93.   Dressler WW, Balieiro MC, Ribeiro RP, Dos Santos JE. Culture and the Immune System: Cultural Consonance in Social Support and C-reactive Protein in Urban Brazil. Medical anthropology quarterly 2016;30:259-77.
94.   Pandey D, Shrivastava P. Mediation effect of social support on the association between hardiness and immune response. Asian journal of psychiatry 2017;26:52-5.
95.   Holt-Lunstad J. Why Social Relationships Are Important for Physical Health: A Systems Approach to Understanding and Modifying Risk and Protection. Annual review of psychology 2018;69:437-58.
96.   Glaser R, Kiecolt-Glaser JK, Malarkey WB, Sheridan JF. The influence of psychological stress on the immune response to vaccines. Annals of the New York Academy of Sciences 1998;840:649-55.
97.   Yang Q, Shu HB. Deciphering the pathways to antiviral innate immunity and inflammation. Advances in immunology 2020;145:1-36.

98. Thomas PD, Goodwin JM, Goodwin JS. Effect of social support on stress-related changes in cholesterol level, uric acid level, and immune function in an elderly sample. The American journal of psychiatry 1985;142:735-7.

99. Baron RS, Cutrona CE, Hicklin D, Russell DW, Lubaroff DM. Social support and immune function among spouses of cancer patients. Journal of personality and social psychology 1990;59:344-52.

100. Theorell T, Blomkvist V, Jonsson H, Schulman S, Berntorp E, Stigendal L. Social support and the development of immune function in human immunodeficiency virus infection. Psychosomatic medicine 1995;57:32-6.

101. Gouin JP, Kiecolt-Glaser JK, Malarkey WB, Glaser R. The influence of anger expression on wound healing. Brain, behavior, and immunity 2008;22:699-708.

102. Suarez EC, Boyle SH, Lewis JG, Hall RP, Young KH. Increases in stimulated secretion of proinflammatory cytokines by blood monocytes following arousal of negative affect: the role of insulin resistance as moderator. Brain, behavior, and immunity 2006;20:331-8.

103. Kiecolt-Glaser JK, Loving TJ, Stowell JR, et al. Hostile marital interactions, proinflammatory cytokine production, and wound healing. Archives of general psychiatry 2005;62:1377-84.

104. Kiecolt-Glaser JK, Glaser R, Cacioppo JT, Malarkey WB. Marital stress: immunologic, neuroendocrine, and autonomic correlates. Annals of the New York Academy of Sciences 1998;840:656-63.

105. Kiecolt-Glaser JK, Wilson SJ. Lovesick: How Couples' Relationships Influence Health. Annual review of clinical psychology 2017;13:421-43.

106. Fredrickson BL, Grewen KM, Algoe SB, et al. Psychological well-being and the human conserved transcriptional response to adversity. PloS one 2015;10:e0121839.

107. Forgiveness and Immune Functioning in People Living With HIV-AIDS. ResearchGate, 2011. (Accessed March 1, 2020, at https://www.researchgate.net/publication/265037569_Forgiveness_and_Immune_Functio ning_in_People_Living_with_HIV-AIDS.)

108. Helliwell JF, Huang H. Comparing the happiness effects of real and on-line friends. PloS one 2013;8:e72754.

109. Hsu HC, Chang WC. Social connections and happiness among the elder population of Taiwan. Aging & mental health 2015;19:1131-7.

110. Sephton SE, Koopman C, Schaal M, Thoresen C, Spiegel D. Spiritual expression and immune status in women with metastatic breast cancer: an exploratory study. The breast journal 2001;7:345-53.

111. Shattuck EC, Muehlenbein MP. Religiosity/Spirituality and Physiological Markers of Health. Journal of religion and health 2018.

112. Hulett JM, Armer JM. A Systematic Review of Spiritually Based Interventions and Psychoneuroimmunological Outcomes in Breast Cancer Survivorship. Integrative cancer therapies 2016;15:405-23.

113. Diener E, Tay L, Myers DG. The religion paradox: if religion makes people happy, why are so many dropping out? Journal of personality and social psychology 2011;101:1278-90.

114. Frey BS. Psychology. Happy people live longer. Science (New York, NY) 2011;331:542-3.

115. Fredrickson BL, Grewen KM, Coffey KA, et al. A functional genomic perspective on human well-being. Proceedings of the National Academy of Sciences of the United States of America 2013;110:13684-9.

116. Matsunaga M, Isowa T, Yamakawa K, et al. Association between perceived happiness levels and peripheral circulating pro-inflammatory cytokine levels in middle-aged adults in Japan. Neuro endocrinology letters 2011;32:458-63.

117. Kok BE, Coffey KA, Cohn MA, et al. How positive emotions build physical health: perceived positive social connections account for the upward spiral between positive emotions and vagal tone. Psychological science 2013;24:1123-32.

118. Hayashi T, Tsujii S, Iburi T, et al. Laughter up-regulates the genes related to NK cell activity in diabetes. Biomedical research (Tokyo, Japan) 2007;28:281-5.

119. Hayashi T, Murakami K. The effects of laughter on post-prandial glucose levels and gene expression in type 2 diabetic patients. Life sciences 2009;85:185-7.

120. Matsuzaki T, Nakajima A, Ishigami S, Tanno M, Yoshino S. Mirthful laughter differentially affects serum pro- and anti-inflammatory cytokine levels depending on the level of disease activity in patients with rheumatoid arthritis. Rheumatology (Oxford, England) 2006;45:182-6.

121. Berk LS, Felten DL, Tan SA, Bittman BB, Westengard J. Modulation of neuroimmune parameters during the eustress of humor-associated mirthful laughter. Alternative therapies in health and medicine 2001;7:62-72, 4-6.

122. Carroll JE, Low CA, Prather AA, et al. Negative affective responses to a speech task predict changes in interleukin (IL)-6. Brain, behavior, and immunity 2011;25:232-8.

123. Cohen F, Kearney KA, Zegans LS, Kemeny ME, Neuhaus JM, Stites DP. Differential immune system changes with acute and persistent stress for optimists vs pessimists. Brain, behavior, and immunity 1999;13:155-74.

124. Segerstrom SC, Taylor SE, Kemeny ME, Fahey JL. Optimism is associated with mood, coping, and immune change in response to stress. Journal of personality and social psychology 1998;74:1646-55.

125. Brydon L, Walker C, Wawrzyniak AJ, Chart H, Steptoe A. Dispositional optimism and stress-induced changes in immunity and negative mood. Brain, behavior, and immunity 2009;23:810-6.

126. Rasmussen HN, Scheier MF, Greenhouse JB. Optimism and physical health: a meta-analytic review. Annals of behavioral medicine : a publication of the Society of Behavioral Medicine 2009;37:239-56.

127. Avvenuti G, Baiardini I, Giardini A. Optimism's Explicative Role for Chronic Diseases. Frontiers in psychology 2016;7:295.

128. Tejero-Fernandez V, Membrilla-Mesa M, Galiano-Castillo N, Arroyo-Morales M. Immunological effects of massage after exercise: A systematic review. Physical therapy in sport : official journal of the Association of Chartered Physiotherapists in Sports Medicine 2015;16:187-92.

129. Koelsch S, Boehlig A, Hohenadel M, Nitsche I, Bauer K, Sack U. The impact of acute stress on hormones and cytokines, and how their recovery is affected by music-evoked positive mood. Scientific reports 2016;6:23008.

130. Koyama M, Wachi M, Utsuyama M, Bittman B, Hirokawa K, Kitagawa M. Recreational music-making modulates immunological responses and mood states in older adults. Journal of medical and dental sciences 2009;56:79-90.

131. Kreutz G, Bongard S, Rohrmann S, Hodapp V, Grebe D. Effects of choir singing or listening on secretory immunoglobulin A, cortisol, and emotional state. Journal of behavioral medicine 2004;27:623-35.

132. Fancourt D, Perkins R, Ascenso S, Carvalho LA, Steptoe A, Williamon A. Effects of Group Drumming Interventions on Anxiety, Depression, Social Resilience and Inflammatory Immune Response among Mental Health Service Users. PloS one 2016;11:e0151136.

133. Bittman BB, Berk LS, Felten DL, et al. Composite effects of group drumming music therapy on modulation of neuroendocrine-immune parameters in normal subjects. Alternative therapies in health and medicine 2001;7:38-47.

134. Chen PJ, Chou CC, Yang L, Tsai YL, Chang YC, Liaw JJ. Effects of Aromatherapy Massage on Pregnant Women's Stress and Immune Function: A Longitudinal, Prospective, Randomized Controlled Trial. Journal of alternative and complementary medicine (New York, NY) 2017;23:778-86.

135. Shor-Posner G, Miguez MJ, Hernandez-Reif M, Perez-Then E, Fletcher M. Massage treatment in HIV-1 infected Dominican children: a preliminary report on the efficacy of massage therapy to preserve the immune system in children without antiretroviral medication. Journal of alternative and complementary medicine (New York, NY) 2004;10:1093-5.

136. Billhult A, Lindholm C, Gunnarsson R, Stener-Victorin E. The effect of massage on immune function and stress in women with breast cancer--a randomized controlled trial. Autonomic neuroscience : basic & clinical 2009;150:111-5.

137. Rapaport MH, Schettler P, Breese C. A preliminary study of the effects of a single session of Swedish massage on hypothalamic-pituitary-adrenal and immune function in normal individuals. Journal of alternative and complementary medicine (New York, NY) 2010;16:1079-88.

138. Ballas D, Dorling D. Measuring the impact of major life events upon happiness. International journal of epidemiology 2007;36:1244-52.

139. Garcia D, Sikstrom S. A collective theory of happiness: words related to the word "happiness" in Swedish online newspapers. Cyberpsychology, behavior and social networking 2013;16:469-72.

140. Ishii H, Nagashima M, Tanno M, Nakajima A, Yoshino S. Does being easily moved to tears as a response to psychological stress reflect response to treatment and the general prognosis in patients with rheumatoid arthritis? Clinical and experimental rheumatology 2003;21:611-6.

141. Younas M, Carrat F, Desaint C, Launay O, Corbeau P. Immune activation, smoking, and vaccine response. AIDS (London, England) 2017;31:171-3.

142. de Heens GL, van der Velden U, Loos BG. Cigarette smoking enhances T cell activation and a Th2 immune response; an aspect of the pathophysiology in periodontal disease. Cytokine 2009;47:157-61.

143. Gaydos J, McNally A, Guo R, Vandivier RW, Simonian PL, Burnham EL. Alcohol abuse and smoking alter inflammatory mediator production by pulmonary and systemic immune cells. American journal of physiology Lung cellular and molecular physiology 2016;310:L507-18.

144. Meadows GG, Zhang H. Effects of Alcohol on Tumor Growth, Metastasis, Immune Response, and Host Survival. Alcohol research : current reviews 2015;37:311-22.

145. Barr T, Helms C, Grant K, Messaoudi I. Opposing effects of alcohol on the immune system. Progress in neuro-psychopharmacology & biological psychiatry 2016;65:242-51.

146. Han L, Ran J, Mak YW, et al. Smoking and Influenza-associated Morbidity and Mortality: A Systematic Review and Meta-analysis. Epidemiology (Cambridge, Mass) 2019;30:405-17.

147. Mora JR, Iwata M, von Andrian UH. Vitamin effects on the immune system: vitamins A and D take centre stage. Nature reviews Immunology 2008;8:685-98.

148. Red grapes, blueberries may enhance immune function. Oregon State University, 2013. (Accessed March 1, 2020, at https://www.sciencedaily.com/releases/2013/09/130917125022.htm.)

149. Xu ML, Kim HJ, Wi GR, Kim HJ. The effect of dietary bovine colostrum on respiratory syncytial virus infection and immune responses following the infection in the mouse. Journal of microbiology (Seoul, Korea) 2015;53:661-6.

150. Wong EB, Mallet JF, Duarte J, Matar C, Ritz BW. Bovine colostrum enhances natural killer cell activity and immune response in a mouse model of influenza infection and mediates intestinal immunity through toll-like receptors 2 and 4. Nutrition research (New York, NY) 2014;34:318-25.

151. Jones AW, Cameron SJ, Thatcher R, Beecroft MS, Mur LA, Davison G. Effects of bovine colostrum supplementation on upper respiratory illness in active males. Brain, behavior, and immunity 2014;39:194-203.

152. Kapusta-Duch J, Kopec A, Piatkowska E, Borczak B, Leszczynska T. The beneficial effects of Brassica vegetables on human health. Roczniki Panstwowego Zakladu Higieny 2012;63:389-95.

153. Wintergerst ES, Maggini S, Hornig DH. Immune-enhancing role of vitamin C and zinc and effect on clinical conditions. Annals of nutrition & metabolism 2006;50:85-94.

154. Schapowal A, Klein P, Johnston SL. Echinacea reduces the risk of recurrent respiratory tract infections and complications: a meta-analysis of randomized controlled trials. Advances in therapy 2015;32:187-200.

155. Lee GY, Han SN. The Role of Vitamin E in Immunity. Nutrients 2018;10.

156. Lee CY, Man-Fan Wan J. Vitamin E supplementation improves cell-mediated immunity and oxidative stress of Asian men and women. The Journal of nutrition 2000;130:2932-7.

157. Vitamin E supplementation enhances immune response in the elderly. Nutrition reviews 1992;50:85-7.

158. Rabe SZ, Ghazanfari T, Siadat Z, Rastin M, Rabe SZ, Mahmoudi M. Anti-inflammatory effect of garlic 14-kDa protein on LPS-stimulated-J774A.1 macrophages. Immunopharmacology and immunotoxicology 2015;37:158-64.

159. Arreola R, Quintero-Fabian S, Lopez-Roa RI, et al. Immunomodulation and anti-inflammatory effects of garlic compounds. Journal of immunology research 2015;2015:401630.

160. Nantz MP, Rowe CA, Muller CE, Creasy RA, Stanilka JM, Percival SS. Supplementation with aged garlic extract improves both NK and gammadelta-T cell function and reduces the severity of cold and flu symptoms: a randomized, double-blind, placebo-controlled nutrition intervention. Clinical nutrition (Edinburgh, Scotland) 2012;31:337-44.

161. Percival SS. Aged Garlic Extract Modifies Human Immunity. The Journal of nutrition 2016;146:433s-6s.
162. Mashhadi NS, Ghiasvand R, Askari G, Hariri M, Darvishi L, Mofid MR. Anti-oxidative and anti-inflammatory effects of ginger in health and physical activity: review of current evidence. International journal of preventive medicine 2013;4:S36-42.
163. Calder PC. Feeding the immune system. The Proceedings of the Nutrition Society 2013;72:299-309.
164. Sales-Campos H, Soares SC, Oliveira CJF. An introduction of the role of probiotics in human infections and autoimmune diseases. Critical reviews in microbiology 2019;45:413-32.
165. Peters VBM, van de Steeg E, van Bilsen J, Meijerink M. Mechanisms and immunomodulatory properties of pre- and probiotics. Beneficial microbes 2019;10:225-36.
166. Azad MAK, Sarker M, Wan D. Immunomodulatory Effects of Probiotics on Cytokine Profiles. BioMed research international 2018;2018:8063647.
167. Abdollahi E, Momtazi AA, Johnston TP, Sahebkar A. Therapeutic effects of curcumin in inflammatory and immune-mediated diseases: A nature-made jack-of-all-trades? Journal of cellular physiology 2018;233:830-48.
168. Kahkhaie KR, Mirhosseini A, Aliabadi A, et al. Curcumin: a modulator of inflammatory signaling pathways in the immune system. Inflammopharmacology 2019;27:885-900.

Acknowledgments

I am grateful to the countless scientists, reporters, philosophers, and authors who have helped me learn the information I share in this book.

I am grateful to my parents, Sahib and Shashi; my in-laws, Vinod and Kusum; my brother, Kishore and Sundeep; my sisters, Sandhya, Rajni, and Smita; our extended family members; my daughters, Gauri and Sia; and my wife, Richa, for showering me with love that sustains me every day.

I am grateful to all my friends and colleagues for their support and love.

I am especially grateful to Arush Chandna for his help in developing this manuscript and the related website immuneresilience.com.

I am grateful to all my students and patients who trust my values and my ability to be of help. You give me strength every single day.

I am grateful to you all for helping build a kinder, happier, and more hopeful world for our planet's children. Thank you.

Amit

About Dr. Sood

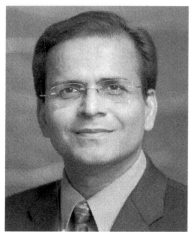

Dr. Amit Sood is married to his lovely wife of 27 years, Dr. Richa Sood. They have two girls, Gauri age 15, and Sia age 9.

Dr. Sood serves as the Executive Director of the Global Center for Resiliency and Wellbeing and The GRIT Institute. Dr. Sood is a former professor of medicine, chair of the Mind-Body Medicine Initiative, and director of student life and wellness at Mayo Clinic.

Dr. Sood completed his residency in internal medicine at the Albert Einstein School of Medicine, an integrative medicine fellowship at the University of Arizona, and earned a master's degree in clinical research from Mayo Clinic College of Medicine. He has received several National Institutes of Health grants and foundation awards to test and implement integrative and mind-body approaches within medicine.

Dr. Sood has developed an innovative approach toward mind-body medicine by incorporating concepts from neuroscience, evolutionary biology, psychology, philosophy, and spirituality. His resulting program, Stress Management and Resiliency Training (SMART©) help patients learn skills to decrease stress and enhance resiliency by improving self-awareness, engagement, and emotional resilience. Interventions adapted from the program reach approximately 50,000 patients and learners each year. The program has been tested in over 30 clinical trials.

Dr. Sood's programs are offered for a wide variety of patients and learners including to improve resiliency; decrease stress and anxiety; enhance well-being and happiness; cancer symptom relief and prevention; and wellness solutions for caregivers, corporate executives, health care professionals, parents, and students. SMART© program is now integrated into several hospitals and health systems for managing burnout, leadership training, for enhancing resilience among nurses, and is being offered with all ages of students, and teachers.

Dr. Sood has authored or co-authored over 70 peer-reviewed articles, and several editorials, book chapters, abstracts, and letters. Dr. Sood is the author of the books *SMART with Dr. Sood, The Mayo Clinic Guide to Stress-Free Living, The Mayo Clinic Handbook for Happiness, Immerse: A 52-Week Course in Resilient Living, Stronger: The Science and Art of Stress Resilience, and Mindfulness Redesigned for the Twenty-First Century.* As an international expert in his field, Dr. Sood's work has been widely cited in the press including – *The Atlantic Monthly, USA Today, Wall Street Journal, New York Times, NPR, Reuters Health, Time Magazine (online), Good Housekeeping, Parenting, Real Simple, Shape, US News, Huffington Post, Men's Health Magazine, The Globe and Mail, CBS News, Fox News, and others.* He has interviewed with several prominent TV and radio shows, both nationally and internationally. He was selected as one of the 2015 Health care pioneers by the Robert Wood Johnson Foundation.

He is a highly sought after speaker and delivered the TEDx talk – *Happy Brain: How to Overcome Our Neural Predispositions to Suffering.* He has mentored several hundred fellows, medical students, instructors, consultants, and residents. Dr. Sood is currently working with several large hospitals and health systems, and Fortune 500 companies to implement his solutions for employee wellbeing. He is currently training about 150 students to become certified resilience trainers through his CeRT (Certified Resilience Trainer) program (resiliencetrainer.com).

Dr. Sood has received several awards for his work, including the Mayo's 2010 Distinguished Service Award, Mayo's 2010 Innovator of the Year Award, Mayo's 2013 outstanding physician scientist award, and was chosen as one among the top 20 intelligent optimists "helping the world be a better place" by *Ode Magazine.*

Dr. Sood serves on the Wellbeing Advisory Board of Everyday Health.

Made in the USA
San Bernardino, CA
16 March 2020